Instant Vortex Easy Cooking

The Instant Vortex Air Fryer Cookbook With Over 50 Delicious Recipes

Zoe Baker

© Copyright 2021 - All rights reserved.

The content contained within this book may not be reproduced, duplicated or transmitted without direct written permission from the author or the publisher.

Under no circumstances will any blame or legal responsibility be held against the publisher, or author, for any damages, reparation, or monetary loss due to the information contained within this book. Either directly or indirectly.

Legal Notice:

This book is copyright protected. This book is only for personal use. You cannot amend, distribute, sell, use, quote or paraphrase any part, or the content within this book, without the consent of the author or publisher.

Disclaimer Notice:

Please note the information contained within this document is for educational and entertainment purposes only. All effort has been executed to present accurate, up to date, and reliable, complete information. No warranties of any kind are declared or implied. Readers acknowledge that the author is not engaging in the rendering of legal, financial, medical or professional advice. The content within this book has been derived from various sources. Please consult a licensed professional before attempting any techniques outlined in this book.

By reading this document, the reader agrees that under no circumstances is the author responsible for any losses, direct or indirect, which are incurred as a result of the use of information contained within this document, including, but not limited to, — errors, omissions, or inaccuracies.

Table of Content

- BREAKFAST 9
- Baked Eggs 10
- Bagels   11
- Toasted Quinoa Chunks 13
- Lime and Cumin Quinoa 14
- Fancy Breakfast Quinoa 15
- Dr. Sebi Kamut Puff Cereal 16
- Fresh Sautéed Apple 17
- Perfect Vegetable Roast 18
- Herb Frittata 19
- SNACK   21
- Apple Dumplings 22
- Apple Pie in Air Fryer 23
- Peanut Butter Banana Bread 24
- Chocolate Banana Bread 26
- Perfect Crispy Potatoes 28
- Allspice Chicken Wings 29
- Friday Night Pineapple Sticky Ribs 30
- Raspberry Cream Roll-Ups 31
- Air Fryer Chocolate Cake 33
- Banana-Choco Brownies 34
- Chocolate Donuts 35
- Easy Air Fryer Donuts 36
- Chocolate Soufflé for Two 37
- Fried Bananas with Chocolate Sauce 38
- Tandoori-Style Chickpeas 39
- Roasted Garlic and Onion Dip 40
- Apple Hand Pies 42
- Chocolaty Banana Muffins 43
- Blueberry Lemon Muffins 45

Cheese-Filled Bread Bowl 46

LUNCH 49

Air Fried Section and Tomato 50
Quick Fry Chicken with Cauliflower and Water Chestnuts 51
Simple Beef Sirloin Roast 53
Seasoned Beef Roast 54
Cheesy Salmon Fillets 55
Tuna Steaks 56
Air-Fried Lean Pork Tenderloin 57
Air Fried Artichoke Hearts 58
Air-Fryer Onion Strings 59
Nana"s Pork Chops with Cilantro 60
Paprika Burgers with Blue Cheese 61
Air Fried Spinach 62
Air Fried Zucchini Blooms 63
Air Fried Salmon Belly 64
Stuffed Portabella Mushrooms 65
Breaded Lean Pork Chops on Spinach Salad 67
Peppery Butter Swordfish Steaks 69

DINNER 72

Grilled Vienna Sausage with Broccoli 73
Aromatic T-bone Steak with Garlic 74
Sausage Scallion Balls 75
Cube Steak with Cowboy Sauce 76
Steak Fingers with Lime Sauce 77
Beef Kofta Sandwich 79
Classic Beef Ribs 80
Spicy Short Ribs with Red Wine Sauce 81
Beef Schnitzel with Buttermilk Spaetzle 83
Beef Sausage Goulash 85
Mom"s Toad in the Hole 87

Beef Nuggets with Cheesy Mushrooms 88
Asian-Style Beef Dumplings 89
Broiled Italian Chicken 91
Asian Style Chicken Meal 92

BREAKFAST

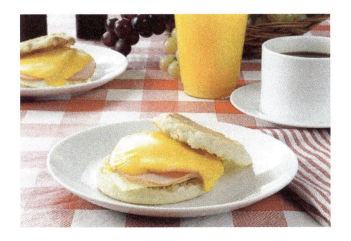

Baked Eggs

Preparation Time: 5 minutes **Cooking Time:** 17 minutes **Servings:** 2 **INGREDIENTS:**

- 2 tablespoons frozen spinach, thawed
- ½ teaspoon salt
- ¼ teaspoon ground black pepper
- 2 eggs, pastured
- 3 teaspoons grated parmesan cheese, reduced-fat
- 2 tablespoons milk, unsweetened, reduced-fat

DIRECTION:

1. Switch on the air fryer, insert fryer basket, grease it with olive oil, then shut with its lid, set the fryer at 330 degrees F and preheat for 5 minutes.
2. Meanwhile, take two silicon muffin cups, grease them with oil, then crack an egg into each cup and evenly add cheese, spinach, and milk.
3. Season the egg with salt and black pepper and gently stir the ingredients, without breaking the egg yolk.
4. Open the fryer, add muffin cups in it, close with its lid and cook for 8 to 12 minutes until eggs have cooked to desired doneness.
5. When air fryer beeps, open its lid, take out the muffin cups and serve.

NUTRITION: Calories 161 Cal Carbs 3 g Fat 11.4 g Protein 12.1 g Fiber 1.1 g

Bagels

Preparation Time: 10 minutes **Cooking Time:** 20 minutes **Servings:** 6 **INGREDIENTS:**

- 2 cups almond flour
- 2 cups shredded mozzarella cheese, low-fat
- 2 tablespoons butter, unsalted
- 1 1/2 teaspoon baking powder
- 1 teaspoon apple cider vinegar
- 1 egg, pastured
- For Egg Wash:
- 1 egg, pastured
- 1 teaspoon butter, unsalted, melted

DIRECTION:

1. Place flour in a heatproof bowl, add cheese and butter, then stir well and microwave for 90 seconds until butter and cheese has melted.
2. Then stir the mixture until well combined, let it cool for 5 minutes and whisk in the egg, baking powder, and vinegar until incorporated and dough comes together.
3. Let the dough cool for 10 minutes, then divide the dough into six pieces, shape each piece into a bagel and let the bagels rest for 5 minutes.
4. Prepare the egg wash and for this, place the melted butter in a bowl, whisk in the egg until blended and then brush the mixture generously on top of each bagel.
5. Take a fryer basket, line it with parchment paper and then place prepared bagels in it in a single layer.
6. Switch on the air fryer, insert fryer, then shut with its lid, set the fryer at 350 degrees F and cook for 10 minutes at the 350 degrees F until

bagels are nicely golden and thoroughly cooked, turning the bagels halfway through the frying.
7. When air fryer beeps, open its lid, transfer bagels to a serving plate and cook the remaining bagels in the same manner.
8. Serve straight away.

NUTRITION: Calories 408.7 Cal   Carbs 8.3 g   Fat 33.5 g Protein 20.3g Fiber 4g

Toasted Quinoa Chunks

Basic Recipe

Preparation Time: 10 minutes **Cooking Time:** 15 minutes **Serving:** 4

INGREDIENTS:

- 8 ounces walnuts
- 1/2 cup uncooked quinoa
- 1 teaspoon salt
- 1 tablespoon olive oil
- 1 teaspoon ground onion powder
- 1 teaspoon paprika powder

DIRECTIONS:

1. Preheat your Air Fryer to 400 degrees F
2. Take a bowl and mix everything
3. Transfer mixture to Air Fryer cooking basket lined with parchment paper
4. Bake it for 10 minutes
5. Break into pieces and serve
6. Enjoy!

NUTRITION: Calories 187 kcal Carbs 6 g Fat 3 g Protein 5 g

Lime and Cumin Quinoa

Intermediate Recipe Preparation Time: 10 minutes **Cooking Time:** 30 minutes **Serving:** 4

INGREDIENTS:

- 2 tablespoons avocado oil
- 1/4 white onion, chopped
- Pinch of salt
- 2 garlic cloves, minced
- 1 cup quinoa
- 1/2 lime, juiced
- 1 tablespoon onion powder
- 1 teaspoon chili powder
- 1/4 teaspoon paprika
- 2 cups Sebi friendly vegetable stock

DIRECTIONS:

1. Preheat your Air Fryer to 300 degrees F
2. Take a pan and place it over medium heat
3. Add onion and salt, Sauté for 3 minutes
4. Add garlic, quinoa, lime, cumin, chili, paprika and Sauté for 2 minutes
5. Transfer mix to Air Fryer cooking basket
6. Add stock and cook for 20-25 minutes
7. Serve and enjoy

NUTRITION: Calories 266 kcal Carbs 40g Fat 8g Protein 9g

Fancy Breakfast Quinoa

Basic Recipe

Preparation Time: 10 minutes **Cooking Time:** 3 Minutes **Serving:** 4

INGREDIENTS:

- 1/2 cup walnuts, soaked and chopped
- 4 ounces sesame seeds, soaked
- 2 ounces hemp seeds, soaked overnight
- 1 teaspoon date sugar
- 1/2 teaspoon ground cinnamon
- 5 ounces quinoa puff
- 1 teaspoon hemp seed oil
- 1 cup of coconut milk

DIRECTIONS:

1. Take a bowl and mix in all the seeds and spices
2. Add hemp seed oil
3. Stir well until the mixture is thick
4. Flatten mixture on your cooking basket
5. Preheat your Air Fryer to 330 degrees F
6. Transfer to your Air fryer and cook for 2-3 minutes until light brown
7. Transfer mix to a serving bowl
8. Add quinoa puff, stir well and add coconut milk stir again
9. Serve and enjoy

NUTRITION: Calories 510 kcal Carbs 50 g Fat 8 g Protein 21g

Dr. Sebi Kamut Puff Cereal

Basic Recipe

Preparation Time: 10 minutes **Cooking Time:** 12 minutes **Serving:** 4

INGREDIENTS:

- Agave nectar
- 6 ounces bag of Kamut puff

DIRECTIONS:

1. Begin by spreading Kamut Puffs over your Air Fryer cooking basket, Drizzle with agave nectar on top
2. Stir well
3. Transfer to Air Fryer and cook for 8-12 minutes
4. Let the puffs cool for 10-15 minutes
5. Enjoy with coconut milk and use it as needed! **NUTRITION:** Calories 196 kcal Carbs 29 g Fat 8 g Protein 2g

Fresh Sautéed Apple

Basic Recipe

Preparation Time: 10 minutes **Cooking Time:** 10 minutes **Serving:** 4

INGREDIENTS:

- 2 tablespoons olive oil
- 3 apples, peeled, cored and sliced
- 1 tablespoon garlic clove, grated
- 1 tablespoon date sugar
- Pinch of salt

Directions:

1. Preheat your Air Fryer 300 degrees F. Add coconut oil to the cooking basket, add remaining ingredients and stir well.
2. Transfer to Air Fryer, cook for 5-10 minutes, making sure to shake the basket occasionally until golden. Serve and enjoy!

NUTRITION: Calories 32 kcal Carbs 32g Fat 9g Protein 3g

Perfect Vegetable Roast

Basic Recipe

Preparation Time: 10 minutes **Cooking Time:** 10 minutes **Serving:** 4

INGREDIENTS:

- 2 cups Roma tomatoes
- 1/2 cup mushrooms halved
- 1 red bell pepper, seeded and cut into bite-sized portions
- 1 tablespoon coconut oil
- 1 tablespoon garlic powder
- 1 teaspoon salt

DIRECTIONS:

1. Preheat your Air Fryer 400 degrees F
2. Take a bowl and add mushrooms, Roma tomatoes, bell pepper, oil, salt, garlic powder and mix well
3. Transfer to Air Fryer cooking basket
4. Cook for 12-15 minutes, making sure to shake occasionally
5. Serve and enjoy once crispy!

NUTRITION: Calories 19 kcal Carbs 19 g Fat 16 g Protein 7g

Herb Frittata

Preparation Time: 10 minutes **Cooking Time:** 25 minutes **Servings:** 4 **INGREDIENTS:**

- 2 tablespoons chopped green scallions
- 1/2 teaspoon ground black pepper
- 2 tablespoons chopped cilantro
- 1/2 teaspoon salt
- 2 tablespoons chopped parsley
- 1/2 cup half and half, reduced-fat
- 4 eggs, pastured
- 1/3 cup shredded cheddar cheese, reduced-fat

DIRECTION:

1. Switch on the air fryer, insert fryer basket, grease it with olive oil, then shut with its lid, set the fryer at 330 degrees F and preheat for 10 minutes.
2. Meanwhile, take a round heatproof pan that fits into the fryer basket, grease it well with oil and set aside until required.
3. Crack the eggs in a bowl, beat in half-and-half, then add remaining ingredients, beat until well mixed and pour the mixture into prepared pan.
4. Open the fryer, place the pan in it, close with its lid and cook for 15 minutes at the 330 degrees F until its top is nicely golden, frittata has set and inserted toothpick into the frittata slides out clean.
5. When air fryer beeps, open its lid, take out the pan, then transfer frittata onto a serving plate, cut it into pieces and serve.

NUTRITION: Calories 141 Cal   Carbs 2 g   Fat 10   g Protein 8 g   Fiber 0 g

SNACK

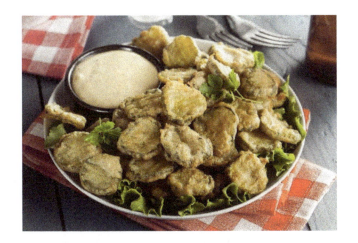

Apple Dumplings

Basic Recipe

Preparation Time: 10 minutes **Cooking Time:** 25 minutes **Servings:** 4 **INGREDIENTS:**

- 2 tbsp. melted coconut oil
- 2 puff pastry sheets
- 1 tbsp. brown sugar
- 2 tbsp. raisins
- 2 small apples of choice

DIRECTIONS:

1. Ensure your air fryer oven is preheated to 356 degrees. Core and peel apples and mix with raisins and sugar. Place a bit of apple mixture into puff pastry sheets and brush sides with melted coconut oil. Place into the air fryer. Cook 25 minutes, turning halfway through. It will be golden when done.

NUTRITION: Calories 367 Fat 7g Protein 2g Sugar: 5g

Apple Pie in Air Fryer

Basic Recipe

Preparation Time: 5 minutes **Cooking Time**: 35 minutes **Serving**: 4 **INGREDIENTS:**

- ½ teaspoon vanilla extract
- 1 beaten egg
- 1 large apple, chopped
- 1 Pillsbury Refrigerator pie crust
- 1 tablespoon butter
- 1 tablespoon ground cinnamon
- 1 tablespoon raw sugar
- 2 tablespoon sugar
- 2 teaspoons lemon juice
- Baking spray

DIRECTIONS:

2. Lightly grease baking pan of air fryer oven with cooking spray. Spread pie crust on bottom of pan up to the sides.
3. In a bowl, mix vanilla, sugar, cinnamon, lemon juice, and apples. Pour on top of pie crust. Top the apples with butter slices. Cover apples with the other pie crust. Pierce with knife the tops of pie.
4. Spread beaten egg on top of crust and sprinkle sugar. Cover with foil.
5. For 25 minutes, cook it on 390°F.
6. Remove foil cook for 10 minutes at 330oF until tops are browned. Serve and enjoy.

NUTRITION: Calories 372 Fat 19g Protein 4.2g Sugar: 5g

Peanut Butter Banana Bread

Intermediate Recipe Preparation Time: 15 minutes **Cooking Time:** 40 minutes **Servings:** 6

INGREDIENTS:

- 1 cup plus 1 tablespoon all-purpose flour
- ¼ teaspoon baking soda
- 1 teaspoon baking powder
- ¼ teaspoon salt
- 1 large egg
- 1/3 cup granulated sugar
- ¼ cup canola oil
- 2 tablespoons creamy peanut butter
- 2 tablespoons sour cream
- 1 teaspoon vanilla extract
- 2 medium ripe bananas, peeled and mashed
- ¾ cup walnuts, roughly chopped

DIRECTIONS:

1. In a bowl and mix the flour, baking powder, baking soda, and salt together.
2. In another large bowl, add the egg, sugar, oil, peanut butter, sour cream, and vanilla extract and beat until well combined.
3. Add the bananas and beat until well combined.
4. Add the flour mixture and mix until just combined.
5. Gently, fold in the walnuts.
6. Place the mixture into a lightly greased pan.
7. Press ―Power Button‖ of Air Fry Oven and turn the dial to select the ―Air Crisp‖ mode.
8. Press the Time button and again turn the dial to set the cooking time to 40

minutes
9. Now push the Temp button and rotate the dial to set the temperature at 330 degrees F.
10. Press ―Start/Pause‖ button to start.
11. When the unit beeps to show that it is preheated, open the lid.
12. Arrange the pan in ―Air Fry Basket‖ and insert in the oven.
13. Place the pan onto a wire rack to cool for about 10 minutes
14. Carefully, invert the bread onto wire rack to cool completely before slicing.
15. Cut the bread into desired-sized slices and serve.

NUTRITION: Calories 384 Fat 23 g Carbs 39.3 g Protein 8.9 g

Chocolate Banana Bread

Basic Recipe

Preparation Time: 15 minutes **Cooking Time:** 20 minutes **Servings:** 8 **INGREDIENTS:**

- 2 cups flour
- ½ teaspoon baking soda
- ½ teaspoon baking powder
- ½ teaspoon salt
- ¾ cup sugar
- 1/3 cup butter, softened
- 3 eggs
- 1 tablespoon vanilla extract
- 1 cup milk
- ½ cup bananas, peeled and mashed
- 1 cup chocolate chips

DIRECTIONS:

1. In a bowl, mix together the flour, baking soda, baking powder, and salt.
2. In another large bowl, add the butter, and sugar and beat until light and fluffy.
3. Add the eggs, and vanilla extract and whisk until well combined.
4. Add the flour mixture and mix until well combined.
5. Add the milk, and mashed bananas and mix well.
6. Gently, fold in the chocolate chips. Place the mixture into a lightly greased loaf pan.
7. Press ―Power Button‖ of Air Fry Oven and turn the dial to select the ―Air Crisp‖ mode.

8. Press the Time button and again turn the dial to set the cooking time to 20 minutes
9. Now push the Temp button and rotate the dial to set the temperature at 360 degrees F.
10. Press ―Start/Pause‖ button to start. When the unit beeps to show that it is preheated, open the lid.
11. Arrange the pan in ―Air Fry Basket‖ and insert in the oven.
12. Place the pan onto a wire rack to cool for about 10 minutes Carefully, invert the bread onto wire rack to cool completely before slicing.
13. Cut the bread into desired-sized slices and serve. **NUTRITION:** Calories 416 Fat 16.5 g Carbs 59.2 g Protein 8.1 g

Perfect Crispy Potatoes

Basic Recipe

Preparation Time: 5 minutes **Cooking Time:** 30 minutes **Servings:** 4 **INGREDIENTS:**

- 1.5 pounds potatoes, halved
- 2 tbsp olive oil
- 3 garlic cloves, grated
- 1 tbsp minced fresh rosemary
- 1 tsp salt
- ¼ tsp freshly ground black pepper

DIRECTIONS:

14. In a bowl, mix potatoes, olive oil, garlic, rosemary, salt, and pepper, until they are well-coated. Arrange the potatoes in the air fryer and cook on 360 F for 25 minutes, shaking twice during the cooking. Cook until crispy on the outside and tender on the inside.

NUTRITION: Calories 365 Fat 13.2 g Carbs 48.6 g Protein 10.1 g

Allspice Chicken Wings

Basic Recipe Preparation Time:

Cooking Time: 45 minutes **Serving:** 8

INGREDIENTS:

- ½ tsp celery salt
- ½ tsp bay leaf powder
- ½ tsp ground black pepper
- ½ tsp paprika
- ¼ tsp dry mustard
    - ¼ tsp cayenne pepper
    - ¼ tsp allspice
    - 2 pounds chicken wings

DIRECTIONS:

15. Grease the air fryer basket and preheat to 340 F. In a bowl, mix celery salt, bay leaf powder, black pepper, paprika, dry mustard, cayenne pepper, and allspice. Coat the wings thoroughly in this mixture.
16. Arrange the wings in an even layer in the basket of the air fryer. Cook the chicken until it's no longer pink around the bone, for 30 minutes then, increase the temperature to 380 F and cook for 6 minutes more, until crispy on the outside.

NUTRITION: Calories 332 Fat 10.1 g Carbs 31.3 g Protein 12 g

Friday Night Pineapple Sticky Ribs

Basic Recipe

Preparation Time: 10 minutes **Cooking Time:** 20 minutes **Servings:** 4 **INGREDIENTS:**

- 2 lb. cut spareribs
- 7 oz salad dressing
- 1 (5-oz) can pineapple juice
- 2 cups water
- Garlic salt to taste
- Salt and black pepper

DIRECTIONS:

17. Sprinkle the ribs with salt and pepper, and place them in a saucepan. Pour water and cook the ribs for 12 minutes on high heat.
18. Dry out the ribs and arrange them in the fryer; sprinkle with garlic salt. Cook it for 15 minutes at 390 F.
19. Prepare the sauce by combining the salad dressing and the pineapple juice. Serve the ribs drizzled with the sauce.

NUTRITION: Calories 316 Fat 3.1 g Carbs 1.9 g Protein 5 g

Raspberry Cream Roll-Ups

Basic Recipe Preparation Time:

Cooking Time:

Serving: 4

INGREDIENTS:

- 1 cup of fresh raspberries, rinsed and patted dry
- ½ cup of cream cheese, softened to room temperature
- ¼ cup of brown sugar
- ¼ cup of sweetened condensed milk
- 1 egg
- 1 teaspoon of corn starch
- 6 spring roll wrappers (any brand will do, we like Blue Dragon or Tasty Joy, both available through Target or Walmart, or any large grocery chain)
- ¼ cup of water

DIRECTIONS:

7. Cover the basket of the air fryer oven with a lining of tin foil, leaving the edges uncovered to allow air to circulate through the basket. Preheat the air fryer oven to 350 degrees.
8. In a mixing bowl, combine the cream cheese, brown sugar, condensed milk, cornstarch, and egg. Beat or whip thoroughly, until all ingredients are completely mixed and fluffy, thick and stiff.
9. Spoon even amounts of the creamy filling into each spring roll wrapper, then top each dollop of filling with several raspberries.
   10. Roll up the wraps around the creamy raspberry filling, and seal the seams with a few dabs of water.
   11. Place each roll on the foil-lined air fryer basket, seams facing down.

12. Set the air fryer oven timer to 10 minutes during cooking; shake the handle of the fryer basket to ensure a nice even surface crisp.
13. After 10 minutes, when the air fryer oven shuts off, the spring rolls should be golden brown and perfect on the outside, while the raspberries and cream filling will have cooked together in a glorious fusion. Remove with tongs and serve hot or cold.

NUTRITION: Calories 351 Fat 20.1g Protein 4.3g Sugar: 5.6g

Air Fryer Chocolate Cake

Basic Recipe

Preparation Time: 5 minutes **Cooking Time:** 35 minutes **Serving:** 8-10 **INGREDIENTS:**

- ½ C. hot water
- 1 tsp. vanilla
- ¼ C. olive oil
- ½ C. almond milk
- 1 egg
- ½ tsp. salt
- ¾ tsp. baking soda
- ¾ tsp. baking powder
- ½ C. unsweetened cocoa powder
- 2 C. almond flour
- 1 C. brown sugar

DIRECTIONS:

1. Preheat your air fryer oven to 356 degrees.
2. Stir all dry ingredients together. Then stir in wet ingredients. Add hot water last.
3. The batter will be thin, no worries.
4. Pour cake batter into a pan that fits into the fryer. Cover with foil and poke holes into the foil.
5. Bake 35 minutes
6. Discard foil and then bake another 10 minutes

NUTRITION: Calories 378 Fat 9g Protein 4g Sugar: 5g

Banana-Choco Brownies

Basic Recipe

Preparation Time: 5 minutes **Cooking Time:** 30 minutes **Servings:** 12 **INGREDIENTS:**

- 2 cups almond flour
- 2 teaspoons baking powder
- ½ teaspoon baking powder
- ½ teaspoon baking soda
- ½ teaspoon salt
- 1 over-ripe banana
- 3 large eggs
- ½ teaspoon stevia powder
- ¼ cup coconut oil
- 1 tablespoon vinegar
- 1/3 cup almond flour
- 1/3 cup cocoa powder

DIRECTIONS:

1. Preheat the air fryer oven for 5 minutes. Combine all ingredients in a food processor and pulse until well-combined.
2. Pour into a baking dish that will fit in the air fryer.
3. Place in the air fryer basket and cook for 30 minutes at 350°F or if a toothpick inserted in the middle comes out clean.

NUTRITION: Calories 75 Fat 6.5g Protein 1.7g Sugar: 2g

Chocolate Donuts

Basic Recipe

Preparation Time: 5 minutes **Cooking Time:** 20 minutes **Servings:** 8-10 **INGREDIENTS:**

- (8-ounce) can jumbo biscuits
- Cooking oil
- Chocolate sauce, such as Hershey's

DIRECTIONS:

4. Separate the biscuit dough into 8 biscuits and place them on a flat work surface. Use a small circle cookie cutter or a biscuit cutter to cut a hole in the center of each biscuit. You can also cut the holes using a knife.
5. Spray the air fryer basket with cooking oil. Place the 4 donuts in the air fryer oven. Do not stack. Spray with cooking oil. Cook for 4 minutes Open the air fryer and flip the donuts. Cook for an additional 4 minutes. Remove the cooked donuts from the air fryer oven, and then repeat for the remaining 4 donuts. Drizzle with chocolate sauce over the donuts and enjoy while warm.

NUTRITION: Calories 181 Fat 98g Protein 3g

Easy Air Fryer Donuts

Basic Recipe

Preparation Time: 5 minutes **Cooking Time:** 10 minutes **Servings:** 8 **INGREDIENTS:**

- Pinch of allspice
- 4 tbsp. dark brown sugar
- ½ - 1 tsp. cinnamon
- 1/3 C. granulated sweetener
- 3 tbsp. melted coconut oil
- 1 can of biscuits

DIRECTIONS:

6. Mix allspice, sugar, sweetener, and cinnamon together.
7. Take out biscuits from can and with a circle cookie cutter, cut holes from centers and place into air fryer.
8. Cook 5 minutes at 350 degrees. As batches are cooked, use a brush to coat with melted coconut oil and dip each into sugar mixture.
9. Serve warm!

NUTRITION: Calories 209 Fat 4g Carbs: 3g Protein 0g

Chocolate Soufflé for Two

Basic Recipe

Preparation Time: 5 minutes **Cooking Time**: 14 minutes **Servings:** 4 **INGREDIENTS:**

- 2 tbsp. almond flour
- ½ tsp. vanilla
- 3 tbsp. sweetener
- 2 separated eggs
- ¼ C. melted coconut oil
- 3 ounces of semi-sweet chocolate, chopped

DIRECTIONS:

1. Brush coconut oil and sweetener onto ramekins.
2. Melt coconut oil and chocolate together.
3. Beat egg yolks well, adding vanilla and sweetener. Stir in flour and ensure there are no lumps.
4. Preheat the air fryer oven to 330 degrees.
5. Whisk egg whites till they reach peak state and fold them into chocolate mixture.
6. Pour batter into ramekins and place into the air fryer oven.
7. Cook 14 minutes
8. Serve with powdered sugar dusted on top.

NUTRITION: Calories 238; Fat 6g Carbs: 4g Protein 1g

Fried Bananas with Chocolate Sauce

Basic Recipe

Preparation Time: 10 minutes **Cooking Time:** 10 minutes **Servings:** 4

Ingredients:

- 1 large egg
- ¼ cup cornstarch
- ¼ cup plain bread crumbs
- 3 bananas, halved crosswise
- Cooking oil
- Chocolate sauce

DIRECTIONS:

1. In a small bowl, beat the egg. In another bowl, place the cornstarch. Place the bread crumbs in a third bowl. Dip the bananas in the cornstarch, then the egg, and then the bread crumbs.
2. Spray the air fryer basket with cooking oil. Place the bananas in the basket and spray them with cooking oil.
3. Cook for 5 minutes Open the air fryer and flip the bananas. Cook for an additional 2 minutes Transfer the bananas to plates.
4. Drizzle with the chocolate sauce over the bananas, and serve.
5. You can make your own chocolate sauce using 2 tablespoons milk and ¼ cup chocolate chips. Heat a saucepan over medium-high heat. Add the milk and stir for 1 to 2 minutes Add the chocolate chips. Stir it for 2 minutes, or until the chocolate has melted.

NUTRITION: Calories 203 Fat 6g Carbs: 3g Protein 3g

Tandoori-Style Chickpeas

Basic Recipe

Preparation Time: 5 minutes **Cooking Time:** 15 minutes **Servings**: 6 **INGREDIENTS:**

- 1 (15-ounce) can chickpeas, dry outed and rinsed
- Cooking oil spray
- 2 teaspoons curry powder
- 1 teaspoon smoked paprika
- 1 teaspoon ground cumin
- ½ teaspoon cayenne pepper

DIRECTIONS:

1. Pat the chickpeas dry with paper towels and put in the air fryer basket.
2. Set or preheat the air fryer to 400°F. Place the basket in the air fryer and roast the chickpeas for 5 minutes
3. Remove the basket and spray the chickpeas with some cooking oil; toss.
4. Return the basket to the air fryer and roast for 8 minutes more, shaking the basket once during cooking time.
5. Meanwhile, in a small bowl combine the curry powder, paprika, cumin, and cayenne pepper.
6. Remove the basket from the air fryer and sprinkle with the spice mixture; toss to coat. Continue roasting for 2 minutes or until the chickpeas are fragrant.
7. Let the chickpeas cool for about 10 minutes, and then serve.

NUTRITION: Calories 72 Protein 4g Fat 1g Carbs 12g

Roasted Garlic and Onion Dip

Basic Recipe

Preparation Time: 10 minutes **Cooking Time:** 30 minutes **Servings:** 6 **INGREDIENTS:**

- 2 heads garlic
- 1 tablespoon olive oil
- 1 (8-ounce) package cream cheese, at room temperature
- ½ cup mayonnaise
- 2 tablespoons heavy (whipping) cream
- ¼ teaspoon sea salt
- 3 scallions, sliced
- 1 tablespoon minced fresh chives

DIRECTIONS:

1. Using a very sharp knife, cut off and discard the top 1 inch of the garlic heads, exposing the cloves. Drizzle with each head with the olive oil.
2. Loosely wrap the garlic heads in aluminum foil and place in the air fryer basket.
3. Set or preheat the air fryer to 400°F. Put the basket in the air fryer and roast the garlic for 20 to 30 minutes, opening one foil packet after 20 minutes to see if the garlic cloves are soft. Continue roasting if needed.
4. Remove the foil packets from the air fryer, unwrap the garlic heads, and let cool on a wire rack for 20 minutes
5. Separate the garlic cloves from the head and remove the papery skins; place the cloves in a medium bowl. Mash together until smooth.
6. Beat the cream cheese with the mayonnaise, heavy cream, and salt until smooth. Beat in the roasted garlic paste until well mixed, and then stir in the scallions and chives. Serve.

NUTRITION: Calories 299 Protein 3g Fat 31g Carbs 3g

Apple Hand Pies

Basic Recipe

Preparation Time: 5 minutes **Cooking Time:** 10 minutes **Servings:** 6 **INGREDIENTS:**

- 15-ounces no-sugar-added apple pie filling
- 1 store-bought crust

DIRECTIONS:

6. Lay out pie crust and slice into equal-sized squares. Place the 2 tbsp. filling into each square and seal crust with a fork. Pour into the Oven rack/basket. Place the Rack on the middle-shelf of the Air fryer oven. Set temperature to 390°F, and set time to 8 minutes until golden in color.

NUTRITION: Calories 278 Fat 10g Carbs: 4g Protein 5g

Chocolaty Banana Muffins

Basic Recipe

Preparation Time: 5 minutes **Cooking Time:** 25 minutes **Servings**: 12 **INGREDIENTS:**

- ¾ cup whole wheat flour
- ¾ cup plain flour
- ¼ cup cocoa powder
- ¼ teaspoon baking powder
- 1 teaspoon baking soda
- ¼ teaspoon salt
- 2 large bananas, peeled and mashed
- 1 cup sugar
- 1/3 cup canola oil
- 1 egg
- ½ teaspoon vanilla essence
- 1 cup mini chocolate chips

DIRECTIONS:

7. In a large bowl, mix together flour, cocoa powder, baking powder, baking soda and salt.
8. In another bowl, add bananas, sugar, oil, egg and vanilla extract and beat till well combined.
9. Slowly, add flour mixture in egg mixture and mix till just combined.
10. Fold in chocolate chips.
11. Preheat the air fryer oven to 345 degrees F. Grease 12 muffin molds.
12. Transfer the mixture into prepared muffin molds and cook for about 20-25 minutes or till a toothpick inserted in the center comes out clean.
13. Remove the muffin molds from Air fryer and keep on wire rack to

cool for about 10 minutes. Carefully turn on a wire rack to cool completely before serving.

NUTRITION: Calories 189 Fat 8.3g Carbs 12.2g Protein 3.4g

Blueberry Lemon Muffins

Basic Recipe

Preparation Time: 5 minutes **Cooking Time:** 10 minutes **Servings**: 12 **INGREDIENTS:**

- 1 tsp. vanilla
- Juice and zest of 1 lemon
- 2 eggs
- 1 C. blueberries
- ½ C. cream
- ¼ C. avocado oil
- ½ C. monk fruit
- 2 ½ C. almond flour s

DIRECTIONS:

14. Mix monk fruit and flour together.
15. In another bowl, mix vanilla, egg, lemon juice, and cream together. Add mixtures together and blend well.
16. Spoon batter into cupcake holders
17. Place in air fryer oven. Bake 10 minutes at 320 degrees, checking at 6 minutes to ensure you don't over bake them.

NUTRITION: Calories 317 Fat 11g Carbs: 5g Protein 3g

Cheese-Filled Bread Bowl

Basic Recipe

Preparation Time: 10 minutes **Cooking Time:** 30 minutes **Servings:** 4 **INGREDIENTS:**

- 1 (6-inch) round loaf bread, unsliced
- 2 tablespoons olive oil
- 6 ounces cream cheese, at room temperature
- ½ cup mayonnaise
- ¼ cup whole milk
- 1 cup shredded Havarti cheese
- 1 cup shredded provolone cheese
- ¼ cup grated Parmesan cheese
- 2 scallions, sliced
- 1 teaspoon Worcestershire sauce

DIRECTIONS:

18. Cut the top 1 inch of the bread off. Use a serrated bread knife to cut around the inside of the loaf, leaving about a 1-inch shell. Be careful not to cut through the bottom. Cut the pieces of bread and the top of the loaf into 1-inch cubes and Drizzle with the olive oil.
19. Set or preheat the air fryer to 375°F. Put the bread cubes in the air fryer basket and Bake it for 5 to 8 minutes, shaking halfway through cooking time, until toasted. Place in a serving bowl. Keep the air fryer set to 375°F.
20. Meanwhile, beat the cream cheese with the mayonnaise and milk until smooth. Stir in the Havarti, provolone, and Parmesan cheeses, scallions, and Worcestershire sauce.
21. Spoon the cheese mixture into the center of the bread shell. Put the filled

bread in the air fryer basket and place the basket in the air fryer. Bake at 375°F for 15 to 20 minutes, stirring the mixture halfway through cooking time, until the cheese is melted and starts to brown on top. Serve with the toasted bread and bread sticks, if desired.

NUTRITION: Calories 514 Protein 17g Fat 42g Carbs 17g

LUNCH

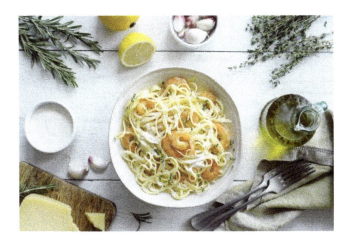

Air Fried Section and Tomato

Intermediate Recipe Preparation Time: 10 minutes **Cooking Time:** 10 minutes **Serving:** 2

INGREDIENTS:

- 1 aubergine, sliced thickly into 4 disks
- 1 tomato, sliced into 2 thick disks
- 2 tsp. feta cheese, reduced Fat
- 2 fresh basil leaves, minced
- 2 balls, small buffalo mozzarella, reduced fat, roughly torn
- Pinch of salt
- Pinch of black pepper

DIRECTIONS:

1. Preheat Air Fryer to 330 degrees F.
2. Spray small amount of oil into the Air fryer basket. Fry aubergine slices for 5 minutes or until golden brown on both sides. Transfer to a plate.
3. Fry tomato slices in batches for 5 minutes or until seared on both sides.
4. To serve, stack salad starting with an aubergine base, buffalo mozzarella, basil leaves, tomato slice, and ½-teaspoon feta cheese.
5. Top of with another slice of aubergine and ½ tsp. feta cheese. Serve.

NUTRITION: Calorie: 140.3 Carbs 26.6 Fat 3.4g Protein 4.2g Fiber 7.3g

Quick Fry Chicken with Cauliflower and Water Chestnuts

Intermediate Recipe Preparation Time: 15 minutes
Cooking Time: 10 minutes **Serving:** 3

INGREDIENTS:

- 1½ pounds chicken thigh fillets, diced
- 1-piece, small red bell pepper, julienned
- 1 piece, thumb-sized ginger, grated
- 2 Tbsp. olive oil
- 1 clove, large garlic, minced
- 2 stalks, large leeks, minced
- 1 can, 5 oz. water chestnuts, quartered
- 1 head, small cauliflower, cut into bite-sized florets
- ¾ cups chicken stock, low sodium
- Seasonings
- 1 tsp. stevia
- 1 Tbsp. fish sauce
- ½ Tbsp. cornstarch, dissolved in
- 4 Tbsp. water
- Pinch of salt
- Pinch of black pepper, to taste
- Garnish:
- Leeks, minced
- 1-piece, large lime, cut into 6 wedges

DIRECTIONS:

1. Preheat Air Fryer to 330 degrees F.

2. Pour olive oil in a pan. Swirl pan to coat. Sauté the garlic, ginger, and leeks for 2 minutes then set aside. Add in water chestnuts, cauliflower, red bell pepper, and chicken broth. Stir well. Cook for 15 minutes.
3. Meanwhile, put the chicken in the Air fryer basket. Fry until seared and golden brown.
4. Add in seasoning into the pan. Stir and cook until the juice thickens.
5. Ladle 1 portion of quick fry veggies and chicken, Garnish with leeks and lemon wedges on the side. Serve.

NUTRITION: Calorie: 220 Carbs 13.6g   Fat 9 Protein 30.5g Fiber 3.8g

Simple Beef Sirloin Roast

Basic Recipe

Preparation Time: 10 minutes **Cooking Time:** 50 minutes **Servings:** 8 **INGREDIENTS:**

- 2½ pounds sirloin roast
- Salt and ground black pepper, as required

DIRECTIONS:

1. Rub the roast with salt and black pepper generously.
2. Insert the rotisserie rod through the roast.
3. Insert the rotisserie forks, one on each side of the rod to secure the rod to the chicken.
4. Arrange the drip pan in the bottom of Instant Vortex Plus Air Fryer Oven cooking chamber.
5. Select ―Roast‖ and then adjust the temperature to 350 degrees F.
6. Set the timer for 50 minutes and press the ―Start‖.
7. When the display shows ―Add Food‖ press the red lever down and load the left side of the rod into the Vortex.
8. Now, slide the rod's left side into the groove along the metal bar so it doesn't move. Then, close the door and touch ―Rotate‖. Press the red lever to release the rod when cooking time is complete.
9. Remove from the Vortex and place the roast onto a platter for about 10 minutes before slicing. With a sharp knife, cut the roast into desired sized slices and serve.

NUTRITION: Calories 201 Fat 8.8 g Carbs 0 g Protein 28.9 g

Seasoned Beef Roast

Basic Recipe

Preparation Time: 10 minutes **Cooking Time:** 45 minutes **Servings:** 10 **INGREDIENTS:**

- 3 pounds beef top roast
- 1 tablespoon olive oil
- 2 tablespoons Montreal steak seasoning

DIRECTIONS:

10. Coat the roast with oil and then rub with the seasoning generously.
11. With kitchen twines, tie the roast to keep it compact. Arrange the roast onto the cooking tray.
12. Arrange the drip pan in the bottom of Instant Vortex plus Air Fryer Oven cooking chamber.
13. Select —Air Fry‖ and then adjust the temperature to 360 degrees F. Set the timer for 45 minutes and press the —Start‖.
14. When the display shows —Add Food‖ insert the cooking tray in the center position.
15. When the display shows —Turn Food‖ do nothing.
16. When cooking time is complete, remove the tray from Vortex and place the roast onto a platter for about 10 minutes before slicing. With a sharp knife, cut the roast into desired sized slices and serve.

NUTRITION: Calories 269 Fat 9.9 g Carbs 0 g Fiber 0 g

Cheesy Salmon Fillets

Intermediate Recipe Preparation Time: 15 minutes
Cooking Time: 10 minutes **Serving**: 3

INGREDIENTS:

- 2 pieces, 4 oz. each salmon fillets, choose even cuts
- ½ cup sour cream, reduced fat
- ¼ cup cottage cheese, reduced Fat
- ¼ cup Parmigiano-Reggiano cheese, freshly grated
- Garnish:
- Spanish paprika
- ½ piece lemon, cut into wedges

DIRECTIONS:

1. Preheat Air Fryer to 330 degrees F.
2. To make the salmon fillets, mix sour cream, cottage cheese, and Parmigiano-Reggiano cheese in a bowl.
3. Layer the salmon fillets in the Air fryer basket. Fry for 20 minutes or until cheese turns golden brown.
4. To assemble, place a salmon fillet and sprinkle paprika. Garnish with lemon wedges and squeeze lemon juice on top. Serve.

NUTRITION: Calorie: 274 Carbs 1g Fat 19g Protein 24g Fiber 0.5g

Tuna Steaks

Intermediate Recipe Preparation Time: 5 minutes **Cooking Time:** 20 minutes **Serving:** 1 **INGREDIENTS:**

- 2 pieces bone-in tuna steaks
- Pinch of salt
- 1 Tbsp. olive oil
- Garnish:
- 1 Tbsp. homemade garlic and parsley butter, divided
- 2 Tbsp. toasted garlic flakes, divided
- ½ small lemons cut into wedges

DIRECTIONS:

1. Preheat Air Fryer to 330 degrees F.
2. Season the tuna steaks with salt.
3. Layer the tuna inside the Air Fryer basket. Fry for 2 minutes on each side. Transfer on a plate.
4. To assemble, place steaks in each plate. Spread parsley and garlic butter. Serve with lemon wedges.

NUTRITION: Calorie: 120 Carbs 0g Fat 1g Protein 27g Fiber 0g

Air-Fried Lean Pork Tenderloin

Intermediate Recipe Preparation Time: 7 minutes **Cooking Time:** 20 minutes **Serving**: 1 **INGREDIENTS:**

- 2 pork tenderloin lean, sliced into matchsticks
- ½ red bell pepper, julienned
- ½ green bell pepper, julienned
- 1 white onion, sliced thinly
- 1 Tbsp. almond flour, finely milled
- 1 tsp. sea salt
    - 1 tsp. ground black pepper
    - ½ tsp. dried pepper flakes

DIRECTIONS:

1. Preheat Air Fryer to 330 degrees F.
2. Season the pork tenderloin with salt, pepper, pepper flakes, and almond flour. Set aside.
3. Layer the pork tenderloin in the Air fryer basket. Cook for 5 minutes or until golden brown.
4. Meanwhile, heat oil in a pan and stir fry onions and bell peppers for 1 minute. To assemble, add cooked pork in a plate and put vegetables on the side. Serve.

NUTRITION: Calorie: 221 Carbs 8g Fat 10g Protein 22g Fiber 0g

Air Fried Artichoke Hearts

Intermediate Recipe Preparation Time: 7 minutes **Cooking Time:** 20 minutes **Serving**: 3

INGREDIENTS:

- 1-pound frozen artichoke hearts, thawed, quartered
- 1-cup plain yogurt, low Fat
- 2 eggs, whisked
- 1 cup almond flour, finely milled
- 1 cup almond flour, coarsely milled
- 1 small lime, sliced into wedges, pips removed
- ½ cup sour cream, reduced Fat
- Pinch of sea salt

DIRECTIONS:

5. Preheat Air Fryer to 330 degrees F.
6. In a bowl, combine yogurt and salt. Soak artichoke hearts for at 15 minutes. Dry out. Discard yogurt. Dredge artichokes in almond flour first, then into eggs, and into coarse-milled almond flour.
7. Layer the artichoke hearts into the Air Fryer basket. Fry for 5 minutes or until golden brown on all sides. Dry out on paper towels. Squeeze lime juice. Serve with lime wedges and sour cream on the side.

NUTRITION: Calorie: 67 Carbs 7g Fat 3g Protein 2g Fiber 1g

Air-Fryer Onion Strings

Intermediate Recipe Preparation Time: 10 minutes **Cooking Time:** 20 minutes **Serving:** 4

INGREDIENTS:

- 2 cups buttermilk
- 1-piece, whole white onion, halved, julienned
- 2 cups almond flour, finely milled
- ½ tsp. cayenne pepper
- Pinch of sea salt
- Pinch of black pepper to taste

DIRECTIONS:

1. Preheat Air Fryer to 330 degrees F.
2. Soak onion strings in buttermilk for 1 hour before frying. Dry out.
3. Meanwhile, mix almond flour, cayenne pepper, salt and pepper in a bowl. Coat onion strings with flour mixture.
4. Layer the onions in Air fryer basket. Fry until golden brown and crisp. Dry out on paper towels. Season it with salt. Serve.

NUTRITION: Calorie: 150 Carbs 13g Fat 17g Protein 2g Fiber 1g

Nana"s Pork Chops with Cilantro

Intermediate Recipe Preparation Time: 5 minutes **Cooking Time:** 20 minutes **Serving:** 6 **INGREDIENTS:**

- 1/3 cup pork rinds
- Roughly chopped fresh cilantro, to taste
- 2 teaspoons Cajun seasonings
- Nonstick cooking spray
- 2 eggs, beaten
- 3 tablespoons almond meal
- 1 teaspoon seasoned salt
- Garlic & onion spice blend, to taste
- 6 pork chops
- 1/3 teaspoon freshly cracked black pepper

DIRECTIONS:

1. Coat the pork chops with Cajun seasonings, salt, pepper, and the spice blend on all sides.
2. Then, add the almond meal to a plate. In a shallow dish, whisk the egg until pale and smooth. Place the pork rinds in the third bowl.
3. Dredge each pork piece in the almond meal; then, coat them with the egg finally, coat them with the pork rinds. Sprits them with cooking spray on both sides.
4. Now, air-fry pork chops for about 18 minutes at 345 degrees F; make sure to taste for doneness after first 12 minutes of cooking. Lastly, garnish with fresh cilantro. Bon appétit!

NUTRITION: 390 Calories 21.3g Fat 1g Carbs 42g Protein

Paprika Burgers with Blue Cheese

Intermediate Recipe Preparation Time: 5 minutes **Cooking Time:** 40Minutes **Serving:** 6

INGREDIENTS:

- 1 cup blue cheese, sliced
- 2 teaspoons dried basil
- 1 teaspoon smoked paprika
    - 2 tablespoons tomato puree
    - 2 small-sized onions, peeled and chopped
    - 1/2 teaspoon ground black pepper
    - 3 garlic cloves, minced
    - 1 teaspoon fine sea salt

DIRECTIONS:

5. Start by preheating your Air Fryer to 385 degrees F.
6. In a mixing dish, combine the pork, onion, garlic, tomato puree, and seasonings; mix to combine well.
7. Form the pork mixture into six patties; cook the burgers for 23 minutes. Pause the machine, turn the temperature to 365 degrees F and cook for 18 more minutes.
8. Place the prepared burgers on a serving platter; top with blue cheese and serve warm.

NUTRITION: 493 Calories 38.6g Fat 4.1g Carbs 30.1g Protein

Air Fried Spinach

Basic Recipe

Preparation Time: 5 minutes **Cooking Time:** 10 minutes **Serving:** 3 **INGREDIENTS:**

- 2½ pounds fresh spinach leaves and tender stems only
- Pinch of sea salt, to taste

DIRECTIONS:

8. Preheat Air Fryer to 330 degrees F. Put spinach in the Air fryer basket. Fry for 20 seconds. Dry out on paper towels. Repeat step with the rest of the spinach. Season it with salt. Serve.

NUTRITION: Calorie: 81.6 Carbs 4.5 Fat 6.9g Protein 1.3g Fiber 1.1g

Air Fried Zucchini Blooms

Basic Recipe

Preparation Time: 5 minutes **Cooking Time:** 10 minutes **Serving:** 3 **INGREDIENTS:**

- 2½ pounds zucchini flowers, rinsed
- 1 cup almond flour, finely milled
- Pinch of sea salt, to taste
- Balsamic vinegar, for garnish

DIRECTIONS:

1. Preheat Air Fryer to 330 degrees F.
2. Half-fill deep fryer with oil. Set this at medium heat. Lightly season zucchini flowers with salt, and then dredge in almond flour.
3. Layer breaded flowers into the Air Fryer basket Fry until golden brown. Dry out on paper towels. Transfer to a plate. Pour balsamic vinegar if using. Serve.

NUTRITION: Calorie: 117 Carbs 8g Fat 8g Protein 1g Fiber 0g

Air Fried Salmon Belly

Intermediate Recipe Preparation Time: 10 minutes **Cooking Time:** 20 minutes **Serving:** 2

INGREDIENTS:

- 1-pound salmon belly, skin on, trimmed, sliced into ¾-inch thick sliver
- 2 Tbsp. almond flour, finely milled
- Pinch of sea salt
- Dip
- ¼ tsp. fresh garlic, minced
- ½ cup coconut or palm vinegar
- ¼ cup white onion, minced
- ¼ tsp. fish sauce
- 1-piece bird's eye chili, deseeded, minced
- Black pepper to taste

DIRECTIONS:

1. Preheat Air Fryer to 330 degrees F.
2. Combine palm vinegar, fish sauce, white onion, bird's eye chili, garlic, and pepper in a small bowl. Set aside. Season salmon belly with the mixture. Roll in almond flour.
3. Layer the fillet in the Air Fryer's basket. Fry for 5 minutes or until golden brown. Dry out on paper towels.
4. Serve with dip or on bed of rice.

NUTRITION: Calorie: 129 Carbs 5.35g Fat 0.8 Protein 11.99g Fiber 0.3g

Stuffed Portabella Mushrooms

Intermediate Recipe Preparation Time: 10 minutes
Cooking Time: 20 minutes **Serving:** 2

INGREDIENTS:

- 2 dozen fresh portabella mushrooms, minced
- 2 tsp. olive oil, add more for drizzling/greasing
- Filling
- 1 tbsp. olive oil
- 1 onion, minced
- 2 garlic cloves, grated
- 3 tbsp. butter, unsalted
- ¼ cup apple cider vinegar
- 2 tbsp. fresh parsley, minced
- ¼ cup roasted cashew nuts, crushed
- ¼-cup cheddar cheese, reduced fat, grated
- ¼ cup parmesan cheese, grated
- pinch of sea salt
- pinch of black pepper to taste

DIRECTIONS:

1. Preheat Air Fryer to 330 degrees F.
2. Meanwhile, in a pan heat the oil. Sauté the onion and garlic for 2 minutes or until translucent and fragrant.
3. Stir in butter, almonds, mushrooms stems, salt, and pepper. Cook for 3 minutes or until mushrooms turn brown in color.
4. Pour vinegar. Cook until the liquid is reduced. Stir in nuts and Parmesan cheese. Allow mixture to cool.
5. Spoon the mixture into mushroom caps. Layer mushrooms in the prepared

baking dish. Place inside the Air fryer basket. Cook for 20 minutes. Serve.

NUTRITION: Calorie: 129 Carbs 5.35g Fat 0.8g Protein 11.99g Fiber 0.3g

Breaded Lean Pork Chops on Spinach Salad

Intermediate Recipe Preparation Time: 40 Minutes **Cooking Time**: 30 minutes **Serving:** 2

INGREDIENTS:

- 2 pieces lean pork chops, pounded ¼-inch thick using a meat mallet
- Breading and seasonings
- 1 egg, whisked
- ½ tsp. Dijon mustard
- ¼ tsp. dried oregano
- ½ cup almond flour, finely milled
- ¼-cup Parmesan cheese
- Pinch of sea salt
- Pinch of black pepper to taste
- Salad
- 6 cups baby spinach leaves, rinsed, spun-dried
- 2 Tbsp. apple cider vinegar
- 1 Tbsp. extra virgin olive oil
- Pinch of sea salt, to taste

DIRECTIONS:

1. Preheat Air Fryer to 330 degrees F.
2. In a bowl, mix egg, oregano, and mustard. Season it with salt and pepper. Marinate pork chops for 30 minutes. Put inside the refrigerator before frying. In another bowl, mix almond flour and Parmesan cheese. Roll pork chops into breading. Layer pork chops in the Air Fryer basket for 5 minutes or until golden brown. Dry out

on paper towels. Put salad ingredients in a salad bowl. Put pork chop slivers. Mix well to combine. Serve.

NUTRITION: Calorie: 165 Carbs 7.15g Fat 9.9g Protein 11.08g Fiber 0.5g

Peppery Butter Swordfish Steaks

Intermediate Recipe Preparation Time: 30 minutes **Cooking Time:** 35 minutes **Serving:** 4

INGREDIENTS:

- Swordfish steaks and seasoning
- 4 pieces swordfish steaks make shallow incisions through skin
- 1/16 tsp. salt
- 1 tsp. olive oil, for greasing
- Peppery Butter
- 2 tsp. butter, unsalted
- ½ tsp. toasted garlic, store-bought
- 1 tsp. fresh parsley, minced
- ½ tsp. mixed dried ground peppercorns
- ½ lime, sliced into 4 equal wedges, for garnish

DIRECTIONS:

9. Preheat the Air Fryer to 400 degrees F.
10. Using a pastry brush, lightly grease four sheets of aluminum foil with olive oil. This will prevent steak from sticking to the foil, while preserving most of its juices.
11. Season the swordfish steaks with salt. Wrap each piece individually in prepared sheets of aluminum foil.
12. Place two steaks into Air Fryer basket. Place double layer rack into the basket. Layer the remaining fish on top.
13. Fry for 10 minutes. Shake contents of basket once midway through.
14. Remove steaks from machine. Place on a plate. Rest the meat for 10 minutes before removing aluminum foil sheets. Place swordfish steaks directly into plates, and Drizzle with in cooking juices.

15. Combine ingredients in a small microwave oven- safe bowl. Microwave for 3 seconds on highest heat until butter softens. Stir well.
16. Top each steak off with equal portions of peppery butter.
17. Squeeze lime juice over fish before eating. **NUTRITION:** Calorie : 140   Carbs 0g Fat 0 Protein 23g Fiber 0g

DINNER

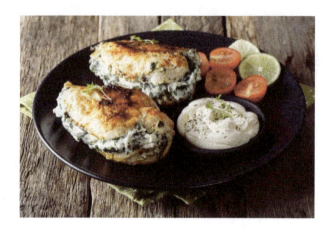

Grilled Vienna Sausage with Broccoli

Basic Recipe

Preparation Time: 5 minutes

Cooking Time: 20 minutes **Servings:** 4

INGREDIENTS:
- 1 pound beef Vienna sausage
- 1/2 cup mayonnaise
- 1 teaspoon yellow mustard
- 1 tablespoon fresh lemon juice
- 1 teaspoon garlic powder
- 1/4 teaspoon black pepper
- 1 pound broccoli

DIRECTIONS:

1. Start by preheating your Air Fryer to 380 degrees F. Spritz the grill pan with cooking oil.
2. Cut the sausages into serving sized pieces. Cook the sausages for 15 minutes, shaking the basket occasionally to get all sides browned. Set aside.
3. In the meantime, whisk the mayonnaise with mustard, lemon juice, garlic powder, and black pepper. Toss the broccoli with the mayo mixture.
4. Turn up temperature to 400 degrees F. Cook broccoli for 6 minutes, turning halfway through the cooking time. Serve the sausage with the grilled broccoli on the side. Bon appétit!

NUTRITION: Calories 477 Fat 43.2g Carbs 7.3g Protein 15.9g

Aromatic T-bone Steak with Garlic

Basic Recipe

Preparation Time: 5 minutes **Cooking Time:** 15 minutes **Servings:** 3 **INGREDIENTS:**

- 1-pound T-bone steak
- 4 garlic cloves, halved
- 1/4 cup all-purpose flour
- 2 tablespoons olive oil
- 1/4 cup tamari sauce
- 2 teaspoons brown sugar
- 4 tablespoons tomato paste
- 1 teaspoon Sriracha sauce
- 2 tablespoons white vinegar
- 1 teaspoon dried rosemary
- 1/2 teaspoon dried basil
- 2 heaping tablespoons cilantro, chopped

DIRECTIONS:

5. Rub the garlic halves all over the T-bone steak. Toss the steak with the flour.
6. Drizzle with the oil all over the steak and transfer it to the grill pan; grill the steak in the preheated Air Fryer at 400 degrees F for 10 minutes
7. Meanwhile, whisk the tamari sauce, sugar, tomato paste, Sriracha, vinegar, rosemary, and basil. Cook an additional 5 minutes
8. Serve garnished with fresh cilantro. Bon appétit! **NUTRITION:** Calories 463 Fat 24.6g Carbs 16.7g Protein 44.7g

Sausage Scallion Balls

Basic Recipe

Preparation Time: 5 minutes **Cooking Time:** 15 minutes **Servings:** 4 **INGREDIENTS:**

- 1 ½ pounds beef sausage meat
- 1 cup rolled oats
- 4 tablespoons scallions, chopped
- 1 teaspoon worcestershire sauce
- Flaky sea salt and freshly ground black pepper, to taste
- 1 teaspoon paprika
- 1/2 teaspoon granulated garlic
- 1 teaspoon dried basil
- 1/2 teaspoon dried oregano
- 4 teaspoons mustard
- 4 pickled cucumbers

DIRECTIONS:

9. Start by preheating your Air Fryer to 380 degrees F. Spritz the Air Fryer basket with cooking oil.
10. In a mixing bowl, thoroughly combine the sausage meat, oats, scallions, Worcestershire sauce, salt, black pepper, paprika, garlic, basil, and oregano.
11. Then, form the mixture into equal sized meatballs using a tablespoon.
12. Place the meatballs in the Air Fryer basket and cook for 15 minutes, turning halfway through the cooking time. Serve with mustard and cucumbers. Bon appétit!

NUTRITION: Calories 560 Fat 42.2g Carbs 21.5g Protein 31.1g

Cube Steak with Cowboy Sauce

Basic Recipe

Preparation Time: 5 minutes **Cooking Time:** 15 minutes **Servings:** 4 **INGREDIENTS:**

- 1 ½ pounds cube steak
- Salt, to taste
- 1/4 teaspoon ground black pepper, or more to taste
- 4 ounces butter
- 2 garlic cloves, finely chopped
- 2 scallions, finely chopped
- 2 tablespoon fresh parsley, finely chopped
- 1 tablespoon fresh horseradish, grated
- 1 teaspoon cayenne pepper

DIRECTIONS:

13. Pat dry the cube steak and season it with salt and black pepper. Spritz the Air Fryer basket with cooking oil. Add the meat to the basket.
14. Cook in the preheated Air Fryer at 400 degrees F for 14 minutes
15. Meanwhile, melt the butter in a skillet over a moderate heat. Add the remaining ingredients and simmer until the sauce has thickened and reduced slightly. Top the warm cube steaks with Cowboy sauce and serve immediately.

NUTRITION: Calories 469 Fat 30.4g Carbs 0.6g Protein 46g

Steak Fingers with Lime Sauce

Basic Recipe

Preparation Time: 5 minutes **Cooking Time:** 15 minutes **Servings:** 4 **INGREDIENTS:**

- 1 ½ pounds sirloin steak
- 1/4 cup soy sauce
- 1/4 cup fresh lime juice
- 1 teaspoon garlic powder
- 1 teaspoon shallot powder
- 1 teaspoon celery seeds
- 1 teaspoon mustard seeds
- Coarse sea salt and ground black pepper, to taste
- 1 teaspoon red pepper flakes
- 2 eggs, lightly whisked
- 1 cup breadcrumbs
- 1/4 cup parmesan cheese
- 1 teaspoon paprika

DIRECTIONS:

16. Place the steak, soy sauce, lime juice, garlic powder, shallot powder, celery seeds, mustard seeds, salt, black pepper, and red pepper in a large ceramic bowl; let it marinate for 3 hours.
17. Tenderize the cube steak by pounding with a mallet; cut into 1-inch strips.
18. In a shallow bowl, whisk the eggs. In another bowl, mix the breadcrumbs, parmesan cheese, and paprika.
19. Dip the beef pieces into the whisked eggs and coat on all sides. Now, dredge the beef pieces in the breadcrumb mixture.

20. Cook at 400 degrees F for 14 minutes, flipping halfway through the cooking time.
21. Meanwhile, make the sauce by heating the reserved marinade in a saucepan over medium heat; let it simmer until thoroughly warmed. Serve the steak fingers with the sauce on the side. Enjoy!

NUTRITION: Calories 471 Fat 26.3g Carbs 13.9g Protein 42.5g

Beef Kofta Sandwich

Basic Recipe

Preparation Time: 5 minutes **Cooking Time:** 25 minutes **Servings:** 4 **INGREDIENTS:**

- 1/2 cup leeks, chopped
- 2 garlic cloves, smashed
- 1-pound ground chuck
- 1 slice of bread, soaked in water until fully tender
- Salt, to taste
- 1/4 teaspoon ground black pepper, or more to taste
- 1 teaspoon cayenne pepper
- 1/2 teaspoon ground sumac
- 3 saffron threads
- 2 tablespoons loosely packed fresh continental parsley leaves
- 4 tablespoons tahini sauce
- 4 warm flatbreads
- 4 ounces baby arugula
- 2 tomatoes cut into slices

DIRECTIONS:

1. In a bowl, mix the chopped leeks, garlic, ground meat, soaked bread, and spices; knead with your hands until everything is well incorporated.
2. Now, mound the beef mixture around a wooden skewer into a pointed-ended sausage.
3. Cook in the preheated Air Fryer at 360 degrees F for 25 minutes
4. To make the sandwiches, spread the tahini sauce on the flatbread; top with the kofta kebabs, baby arugula and tomatoes. Enjoy!

NUTRITION: Calories 436 Fat 20.5g Carbs 32g Protein 33.7g

Classic Beef Ribs

Basic Recipe

Preparation Time: 5 minutes **Cooking Time:** 30 minutes **Servings:** 4 **INGREDIENTS:**

- 2 pounds beef back ribs
- 1 tablespoon sunflower oil
- 1/2 teaspoon mixed peppercorns, cracked
- 1 teaspoon red pepper flakes
- 1 teaspoon dry mustard
- Coarse sea salt, to taste

DIRECTIONS:

22. Trim the excess fat from the beef ribs. Mix the sunflower oil, cracked peppercorns, red pepper, dry mustard, and salt.
23. Rub over the ribs.
24. Cook in the preheated Air Fryer at 395 degrees F for 11 minutes
25. Turn the heat to 330 degrees F and continue to cook for 18 minutes more. Serve warm.

NUTRITION: Calories 532 Fat 39g Carbs 0.4g Protein 44.7g

Spicy Short Ribs with Red Wine Sauce

Basic Recipe

Preparation Time: 5 minutes **Cooking Time:** 15 minutes **Servings:** 4 **INGREDIENTS:**

- 1 ½ pounds short rib
- 1 cup red wine
- 1/2 cup tamari sauce
- 1 lemon, juiced
- 1 teaspoon fresh ginger, grated
- 1 teaspoon salt
- 1 teaspoon black pepper
- 1 teaspoon paprika
- 1 teaspoon chipotle chili powder
- 1 cup ketchup
- 1 teaspoon garlic powder
- 1 teaspoon cumin

DIRECTIONS:

26. In a ceramic bowl, place the beef ribs, wine, tamari sauce, lemon juice, ginger, salt, black pepper, paprika, and chipotle chili powder.
27. Cover and let it marinate for 3 hours in the refrigerator.
28. Discard the marinade and add the short ribs to the Air Fryer basket. Cook in the preheated Air fry at 380 degrees F for 10 minutes, turning them over halfway through the cooking time.
29. In the meantime, heat the saucepan over medium heat; add the reserved marinade and stir in the ketchup, garlic powder, and cumin.
30. Cook until the sauce has thickened slightly.
31. Pour the sauce over the warm ribs and serve immediately. Bon appétit!

NUTRITION: Calories 505 Fat 31g Carbs 22.1g Protein 35.2g

Beef Schnitzel with Buttermilk Spaetzle

Basic Recipe

Preparation Time: 5 minutes **Cooking Time:** 15 minutes **Servings:** 2 **INGREDIENTS:**

- 1 egg, beaten
- 1/2 teaspoon ground black pepper
- 1 teaspoon paprika
- 1/2 teaspoon coarse sea salt
- 1 tablespoon ghee, melted
- 1/2 cup tortilla chips, crushed
- 2 thin-cut minute steaks
- Buttermilk Spaetzle:
- 2 eggs
- 1/2 cup buttermilk
- 1/2 cup all-purpose flour
- 1/2 teaspoon salt

DIRECTIONS:

32. Start by preheating your Air Fryer to 360 degrees F.
33. In a shallow bowl, whisk the egg with black pepper, paprika, and salt.
34. Thoroughly combine the ghee with the crushed tortilla chips and coarse sea salt in another shallow bowl.
35. Using a meat mallet, pound the schnitzel to 1/4- inch thick.
36. Dip the schnitzel into the egg mixture; then, roll the schnitzel over the crumb mixture until coated on all sides.
37. Cook for 13 minutes in the preheated Air Fryer.
38. To make the spaetzle, whisk the eggs, buttermilk, flour, and salt in a bowl. Bring a large saucepan of salted water to a boil.

39. Push the spaetzle mixture through the holes of a potato ricer into the boiling water; slice them off using a table knife. Work in batches.
40. When the spaetzle float, take them out with a slotted spoon. Repeat with the rest of the spaetzle mixture.
41. Serve with warm schnitzel. Enjoy!

NUTRITION: Calories 522 Fat 20.7g Carbs 17.1g Protein 62.2g

Beef Sausage Goulash

Basic Recipe

Preparation Time: 5 minutes **Cooking Time:** 35 minutes **Servings:** 2 **INGREDIENTS:**

- 1 tablespoon lard, melted
- 1 shallot, chopped
- 1 bell pepper, chopped
- 2 red chilies, finely chopped
- 1 teaspoon ginger-garlic paste
- Sea salt, to taste
- 1/4 teaspoon ground black pepper
- 4 beef good quality sausages, thinly sliced
- 2 teaspoons smoked paprika
- 1 cup beef bone broth
- 1/2 cup tomato puree
- 2 handfuls spring greens, shredded

DIRECTIONS:

42. Melt the lard in a Dutch oven over medium-high flame; sauté the shallots and peppers about 4 minutes or until fragrant.
43. Add the ginger-garlic paste and cook an additional minute. Season it with salt and black pepper and transfer to a lightly greased baking pan.
44. Then, brown the sausages, stirring occasionally, working in batches. Add to the baking pan.
45. Add the smoked paprika, broth, and tomato puree. Lower the pan onto the Air Fryer basket. Bake at 325 degrees F for 30 minutes
46. Stir in the spring greens and cook for 5 minutes more or until they wilt. Serve over the hot rice if desired. Bon appétit!

NUTRITION: Calories 565 Fat 47.1g Carbs 14.3g Protein 20.6g

Mom"s Toad in the Hole

Basic Recipe

Preparation Time: 5 minutes **Cooking Time:** 40 minutes **Servings:** 4 **INGREDIENTS:**

- 6 beef sausages
- 1 tablespoon butter, melted
- 1 cup plain flour
- A pinch of salt
- 2 eggs
- 1 cup semi-skimmed milk

DIRECTIONS:

47. Cook the sausages in the preheated Air Fryer at 380 degrees F for 15 minutes, shaking halfway through the cooking time.
48. Meanwhile, make up the batter mix.
49. Tip the flour into a bowl with salt; make a well in the middle and crack the eggs into it. Mix with an electric whisk; now, slowly and gradually pour in the milk, whisking all the time.
50. Place the sausages in a lightly greased baking pan. Pour the prepared batter over the sausages.
51. Cook in the preheated Air Fryer at 370 degrees F approximately 25 minutes, until golden and risen. Serve with gravy if desired. Bon appétit!

NUTRITION: Calories 584 Fat 40.2g Carbs 29.5g Protein 23.4g

Beef Nuggets with Cheesy Mushrooms

Basic Recipe

Preparation Time: 5 minutes **Cooking Time:** 20 minutes **Servings:** 4 **INGREDIENTS:**

- 2 eggs, beaten
- 4 tablespoons yogurt
- 1 cup tortilla chips, crushed
- 1 teaspoon dry mesquite flavored seasoning mix
- Coarse salt and ground black pepper, to taste
- 1/2 teaspoon onion powder
- 1-pound cube steak, cut into bite-size pieces
- 1-pound button mushrooms
- 1 cup Swiss cheese, shredded

DIRECTIONS:

52. In a shallow bowl, beat the eggs and yogurt. In a resealable bag, mix the tortilla chips, mesquite seasoning, salt, pepper, and onion powder.
53. Dip the steak pieces in the egg mixture; then, place in the bag, and shake to coat on all sides.
54. Cook at 400 degrees F for 14 minutes, flipping halfway through the cooking time.
55. Add the mushrooms to the lightly greased cooking basket. Top with shredded Swiss cheese.
56. Bake in the preheated Air Fryer at 400 degrees F for 5 minutes Serve with the beef nuggets. Bon appétit!

NUTRITION: Calories 355 Fat 15.7g Carbs 13.6g Protein 39.8g

Asian-Style Beef Dumplings

Basic Recipe

Preparation Time: 5 minutes **Cooking Time:** 20 minutes **Servings**: 5 **INGREDIENTS:**

- 1/2-pound ground chuck
- 1/2-pound beef sausage, chopped
- 1 cup Chinese cabbage, shredded
- 1 bell pepper, chopped
- 1 onion, chopped
- 2 garlic cloves, minced
- 1 medium-sized egg, beaten
- Sea salt and ground black pepper, to taste
- 20 wonton wrappers
- 2 tablespoons soy sauce
- 2 teaspoons sesame oil
- 2 teaspoons sesame seeds, lightly toasted
- 2 tablespoons seasoned rice vinegar
- 1/2 teaspoon chili sauce

DIRECTIONS:

1. To make the filling, thoroughly combine the ground chuck, sausage, cabbage, bell pepper, onion, garlic, egg, salt, and black pepper. Place the wrappers on a clean and dry surface. Now, divide the filling among the wrappers.
2. Then, fold each dumpling in half and pinch to seal. Transfer the dumplings to the lightly greased cooking basket. Bake at 390 degrees F for 15 minutes, turning over halfway through.
3. In the meantime, mix the soy sauce, sesame oil, sesame seeds, rice vinegar, and chili sauce. Serve the beef dumplings with the sauce on the side. Enjoy!

NUTRITION: Calories; 353 Fat; 16.7g Carbs; 29.5g Protein; 23.1g

Broiled Italian Chicken

Basic Recipe

Preparation Time: 5-10 minutes **Cooking Time:** 20 minutes **Servings:** 4

INGREDIENTS:

- ¾ cup shredded parmesan
- 1 cup panko breadcrumbs
- 4 chicken thighs with bone and skin
- 2 eggs, large
- 1 teaspoon Italian seasoning
- ½ teaspoon ground black pepper
- 1 teaspoon garlic powder
- ½ teaspoon kosher salt

DIRECTIONS:

57. Rub black pepper and salt over the chicken. In a mixing bowl, combine the panko breadcrumbs, Italian seasoning, garlic powder, and parmesan.
58. Beat the eggs in another bowl. Coat the chicken first with the egg, then with the crumb mixture.
59. Place Instant Pot Air Fryer Crisp over kitchen platform. Press Air Fry, set the temperature to 400°F and set the timer to 5 minutes to preheat. Press —Start‖ and allow it to preheat for 5 minutes.
60. In the inner pot, place the Air Fryer basket. In the basket, add the chicken.
61. Close the Crisp Lid and press the —Broil‖ setting. Set temperature to 400°F and set the timer to 20 minutes. Press —Start.‖ No need to flip in between.
62. Open the Crisp Lid after cooking time is over. Serve warm.

NUTRITION: Calories 577 Fat 32g Carbs 14g Protein 42g

Asian Style Chicken Meal

Basic Recipe

Preparation Time: 5-10 minutes **Cooking Time:** 30 minutes **Servings:** 2-3 **INGREDIENTS:**

- ¼ cup honey
- ½ cup rice vinegar
- 1-pound chicken wings
- 1 teaspoon sea salt
- 2 cloves garlic, minced
- 1 teaspoon ginger, grated
- 1 small orange, zest, and juice
- 2 teaspoons red chili pepper paste

DIRECTIONS:

63. Place Instant Pot Air Fryer Crisp over kitchen platform. In the inner pot, add 2 cups water and arrange trivet and place the chicken wings over.
64. Close the Pressure Lid and press the —Pressure‖ setting. Set the —Hi‖ pressure level and set the timer to 2 minutes. Press —Start.‖ Instant Pot will start building pressure. Quick-release pressure after cooking time is over (just press the button on the lid), and open the lid. Take out the wings and empty water.
65. In a mixing bowl, combine the orange zest, orange juice, rice vinegar, honey, red pepper paste, ginger, garlic, and salt.
66. Add the sauce in the pot and place trivet; place the chicken over the trivet.
67. Close the Crisp Lid and press the —Air Fry‖ setting. Set temperature to 390°F and set the timer to 30 minutes. Press —Start.‖

68. Halfway down, open the Crisp Lid, shake the basket and close the lid to continue cooking for the remaining time.
69. Open the Crisp Lid after cooking time is over. Serve the chicken with the honey sauce.

NUTRITION: Calories 448 Fat 17g Carbs 41g Protein 24g

CPSIA information can be obtained
at www.ICGtesting.com
Printed in the USA
BVHW010836230421
605389BV00017B/434